CBD & Hemp Oil

Ryan Timmons

© Copyright 2019 by Ryan Timmons - All rights reserved.

The following Book is reproduced below with the goal of providing information that is as accurate and reliable as possible. Regardless, purchasing this Book can be seen as consent to the fact that both the publisher and the author of this book are in no way experts on the topics discussed within and that any recommendations or suggestions that are made herein are for entertainment purposes only. Professionals should be consulted as needed prior to undertaking any of the action endorsed herein.

This declaration is deemed fair and valid by both the American Bar Association and the Committee of Publishers Association and is legally binding throughout the United States.

Furthermore, the transmission, duplication, or reproduction of any of the following work including specific information will be considered an illegal act irrespective of if it is done electronically or in print. This extends to creating a secondary or tertiary copy of the work or a recorded copy and is only allowed with the express written consent from the Publisher. All additional right reserved.

The information in the following pages is broadly considered a truthful and accurate account of facts and as such, any inattention, use, or misuse of the information in question by the reader will render any resulting actions solely under their purview. There are no scenarios in which the publisher or the original author of this work can be in any fashion deemed liable for any hardship or damages that may befall them after undertaking information described herein.

Additionally, the information in the following pages is intended only for informational purposes and should thus be thought of as universal. As befitting its nature, it is presented without assurance regarding its prolonged validity or interim quality. Trademarks that are mentioned are done without written consent and can in no way be considered an endorsement from the trademark holder.

Contents

Introduction 1

What is CBD and Hemp Oil? 3

What is CBD oil? 4

What is hemp oil? 7

What is the difference between CBD and hemp? 9

What is THC 10

The science behind CBD oil and how it helps heal the body 16

How is CBD different from marijuana? 19

Is it safe for me to use? 21

Are there any effects of using CBD and hemp oil? 24

How long does it take to feel the effects? 26

How long do the effects last? 28

How CBD Can Help Alleviate Your Aches and Pains 30

How can CBD oil help reduce inflammation 32

Depression and Anxiety 36

Using CBD oil to help with depression............... 36

How can CBD help with Anxiety?....................... 39

Other Health Benefits 43

Cancer and chemotherapy 45

Diabetes and heart disease................................... 49

Muscle spasms and seizures................................. 50

Autoimmune disorders 52

Fibromyalgia... 53

Post-traumatic stress disorder............................... 54

Can be used to help with weight loss.................. 56

The Essentials to Know When Buying CBD Oils 58

How do I know when I am getting a product that is high quality? 59

What concentration of CBD should be in the product?.. 63

How do I know that the oil is pure and potent? 64

How much should I spend on the product?........ 65

How do I find a good supplier? 66

Consumption.. 68

Different methods of consuming CBD oil............68

Should I take it with food?......................76

The best time of day to take? 77

What dosage should I take 77

Things to consider when taking CBD for the first time..80

The Different Strains of CBD 82

Hemp Oils..88

Cannabis use, without having to worry about the high..90

CBD doesn't show up in hemp seed oil 92

Methods of getting the CBD out of the hemp 94

Side Effects 97

Will I experience any side effects? 98

How will I know I am having a negative reaction?
....101

Should I see a doctor before starting?................104

Do medications and CBD oils mix? 105

Myths and Mistakes...............................110

Common myths about CBD oil 111

Mistakes you should avoid when taking this oil? 117

Legality of CBD Oil 125

Are CBD and hemp oils legal? 125

Can I fail a drug test taking CBD oil? 132

Is it legal to grow and make your own CBD oil? 134

Is it legal to sell? 135

Conclusion 138

Description 139

Introduction

Congratulations on downloading CBD and Hemp Oil and thank you for doing so. The only thing I ask is if you could please leave an honest review after finishing this book, thanks

In the following chapters we will discuss everything that you need to know to get started with using CBD oil in your own life. While marijuana is only legal in certain states right now, the CBD, which comes from the same part of the plant, is a substance that can really give you a ton of great benefits, without the issue of getting high or any of the negative side effects. This guidebook is going to take a look at CBD oil and hemp oil and why it is something you should consider in your own life.

In this guidebook, we will dive into some of the basics of CBD oil, such as what it is and why it has become so popular. We will then explore some of the many health benefits that you can expect when you decide to add this treatment into your routine. From dealing with headaches to joint pain to fighting off cancer, inflammation, and so much more, CBD oil may be the solution you didn't know you were looking for.

From here, we will explore some of the specifics that you need to know to start taking this kind of oil. We will look at the recommended dosage for each condition, the best time of day to take this oil, and even the different methods you can use to ingest the oil. We will also look at some of the legality of using and selling the oil, the biggest mistakes that beginners make when they start, and so much more.

There are so many benefits that you can receive when you first get started with CBD oil. Whether you have been dealing with some of these common ailments for a long time, or you are pretty healthy as a whole but just want to feel even better, then CBD could be a major help in your life. Make sure to check out this guidebook to help you get started!

There are plenty of books about this subject on the market, so thanks again for choosing this one! Every effort was made to ensure it is full of as much useful information as possible. Enjoy!

Chapter 1

What is CBD and Hemp Oil?

Perhaps you have heard rumors of CBD oil. You may have heard that it has the power to help with almost any ailment and illness out there. You may have heard that it is more effective at reducing aches and pains, and even fighting off cancer than many other common medications on the market that usually come with negative side effects. Maybe you are suffering from some negative health issues yourself, and you want to be able to effectively deal with it, while other options have failed.

In this chapter, we are going to take a look at some of the information that you will need to know to help better your understanding of CBD and hemp oil. We will look at what each of these are, why they are so important, and some of the ways that they can work in your body to improve your health.

What is CBD oil?

Cannabidiol oil, or CBD oil, is an oil that is made from certain strains of a cannabis plant that is naturally low in Tetrahydrocannabinol, commonly known as THC. This is something we will discuss more about later in this book, but THC is a substance found in marijuana plants and is the part that will give the user a high. CBD oil contains only trace amounts of this chemical, and instead, it will be high in cannabinoids, which is also a type of chemical that is found in cannabis plants.

Cannabis is a plant that has been used in many parts of the world for thousands of years. It has long been known for its effectiveness at treating disease and illnesses. However, in the Western world, there has been a change of heart with this plant and all forms of cannabis. It seems to be that the tides may be shifting when it comes to this, and as this status starts to change more, the stigma will also lift, and more and more people will begin to turn towards this oil to give them the treatment they need for their very best health.

The cannabinoids that are found in the CBD oil are healthy and good for the body. The human body is also able to produce some of these substances as well, and there are already many receptors through the body to take on these cannabinoids and use them properly.

These cannabinoids already play a huge role in the body because the endocannabinoid system is known to regulate homeostasis, or a general state of balance in the body. Because of this, this substance is able to regulate and impact different parts of the body such as your response to pain, your immune response, hormone regulation, appetite, sleep, and even your mood.

It has only been recently that science has been able to take a closer look at this and its effects on human health, which means that we are likely to have just scratched the surface on all the cool things that CBD oil can do for your health.

Until recently, the best-known compound that came from the cannabis plant was THC because it is the most active ingredient found in marijuana.

Marijuana actually contains both CBD and THC, but these compounds are found in different amounts in marijuana causing different affects

THC is so well-known because it has the ability to make the user feel high by influencing the way the mind works. This happens whenever the THC is broken down with the use of heat and then introduced into the body, such as when you cook the foods or smoke the plant.

While THC is known to be psychoactive, the CBD is not that way. This means that while you are able to get some great changes to the body and enjoy some medical benefits from using CBD, it is not capable of changing the state of mind of whoever is using it. Most of the time, if CBD is going to be used in a medicinal manner, it is going to be found in the least processed form of the plant, which is called hemp. Hemp and marijuana both come from the same plant, cannabis sativa, but they are actually really different.

This guidebook will spend time looking more into CBD oil and some of the great benefits that it can help you with. There are just so many and as the legal status of this oil begins to change, and more research can be done, both over the short term and the long term, it is likely that we will encounter even more amazing things this oil can help out with.

What is hemp oil?

Hemp oil, which is also known as hempseed oil, is an oil that is obtained by a supplier when they press hemp seeds. When it is done through cold pressing, the hemp oil is going to be either dark or clear light green in color, and it comes in a nutty type of flavor. The darker you are able to get the color, the grassier the flavoring you get to enjoy. This type of oil should never be confused with hash oil, which is a THC containing oil that comes from the cannabis flower.

Refined hemp oil is clear and will lack color, with very little flavor to it. It also lacks the antioxidants and natural vitamins that some claim that it has. This kind of oil is going to be used for many products that deal with body care. But when we talk about industrial hempseed oil, you will find that it is used in plastics, fuel, inks, paints, and lubricants. It can also be used to help produce detergents, shampoos, and soaps.

This oil is going to be produced from varieties of the cannabis sativa that don't have a significant amount of THC, which is the psychoactive elements that are so well-known and loved from the cannabis plant. The process to manufacture this will include cleaning the seed to 99.99 percent, and then the oil will be pressed out of the see. There isn't going to be any THC inside this seed, though it is possible that a tiny bit can end up in the oil if some of the plant matter sticks to the seed during the manufacturing process.

Since 1998, the production of this kind of oil, especially in Canada, has been able to reduce the amount of THC that shows up in the oil. This helps you to get the nutritional value of the hemp oil without having to worry about THC and some of the negative things that may show up with it.

What is the difference between CBD and hemp?

While these two oils may seem similar, and they are going to be able to help the body with some similar benefits, there are a few differences. To start, the seeds of hemp plants are going to be deficient when it comes to CBD levels. In fact, these levels are usually low enough that the hemp oil is not going to be able to produce the same medical benefits as the CBD oil.

In addition, unlike what can be seen with CBD oil, hemp oil is going to have higher levels of the polyunsaturated fats. In fact, this can come in at about 30 percent and will include fatty acids like Omega-3's and Omega-6s. These hemp oils are going to also include vitamin E, which can take up 25 percent of the protein that is found in this kind of oil. This vitamin E can be great for helping you to fight off any free radicals that may be in the body which can balance the hormones, keeps cholesterol levels in line, and can contribute to healthy skin.

The biggest difference in hemp oil and CBD oil is the nutrient density. Most of the benefits that you are going to get from hemp oil come from the high concentration of healthy nutrients, including the ones that we talked about before. These nutrients will enter the body and then produce lower cholesterol and blood pressure readings, reduce diabetes, and can also make your skin shine. But the benefits come from the nutrients and vitamins, not from the cannabinoids that are in them or the way they work with the receptors of the body.

With CBD, you are introducing chemicals into the body that can effectively and positively work with the receptors within your body. They can directly stimulate these receptors in order to ensure that the nervous system does the job it is supposed to do efficiently. This is a direct result of the cannabinoids being able to affect the receptors and not the vitamins and minerals that are found in the oil.

What is THC

As we go through this guidebook, you are going to hear a lot about how CBD oil is low in THC content.

But what exactly is THC and why is it such a good thing that these oils are low in concentration for this chemical. THC, or tetrahydrocannabinol, is a chemical that is found in cannabis and it is the one that is going to cause the euphoric high that marijuana consumers are looking for.

To keep things simple, THC is going to work by binding together the cannabinoid receptors in the nervous system and the brain in order to produce the feelings of being high or being intoxicated. But does this really mean that our bodies have found a way to evolve to use cannabis?

This isn't quite what we mean here. Before you see the relationship between humans and cannabis as symbiotic, it is important to understand that the body can actually produce some of its own cannabinoids. These are seen when it comes to getting a natural high, such as feeling a wave of euphoria after you get done with a good workout or even a successful job. This could be what we experience when there is a runner's high.

What this means is that the human body has been evolved to work well with some of the natural cannabinoids that it releases on its own. But this same system is in place when it comes to taking in THC and some of the other cannabinoids. The body wasn't made to necessarily do well with these cannabinoids, but since it has a system in place that deals with the natural ones that are produced in the body, it is going to use the same system when THC is consumed.

THC is seen as a completely different chemical compound from CBD and hemp, even though they are found in the same plant. The THC can often lead to a number of negative side effects, which is a major reason why it is kept to low concentrations when you consume CBD oil. Some of the common issues that can come up with long-term use of THC (such as what marijuana users may experience) include the following:

Changes to the anatomy of the brain

In some recent studies, there has been a link found between frequent consumption of THC, and alterations to the brain in the corpus callosum. This region of the brain is going to connect the two hemispheres of the brain. Using data from self-reporting of the participants on how much cannabis they used, the researchers were able to find that consumers who took in higher potency strains of THC on a daily basis saw a significant difference in the corpus callosum compared to those who just had THC products on occasion or those who never consumed cannabis at all.

Despite this, the anatomical differences that were seen between those who were frequent users of cannabis with THC and the other groups weren't linked back to psychosis, even though that was something that the researchers had considered. It is important to also take a look at the point that the participants were allowed to self-support how much they consumed, which could change up how accurate the results where.

Bronchitis

Because of the general risk of smoking, whether it is just regular cigarettes or form marijuana, it is possible that the user could develop severe cases of bronchitis. This is why other methods of consumption have gained in popularity and why vaping is a good option.

Memory

A study that was done in 2016 that suggested that there could be a decrease in verbal cognitive function when the THC containing cannabis consumption occurred over a longer period of time. For every five years of using this kind of product, participants would lose memory of one word from a list of 15 words. This is a significant amount, though the study was done on a small sample size of individuals that used THC cannabis over the long term, so it is hard to know how conclusive these findings were.

Psychosis

This one is going to be a big issue only on those who are already predisposed to certain psychotic conditions. These individuals will often see the onset of their symptoms about three years earlier on average if they are already predisposed to these conditions when they use cannabis on a regular basis.

Tolerance to THC

The body is going to slowly build up a tolerance to the THC, especially when you use it in higher levels and over the long term. This promotes more of the negative side effects that are listed above. The downside to this is that when you build up the tolerance to THC is that you will then have increased levels of consumption that comes with these products just to get the desired effects that you want from using the product.

Because of these negative effects, it is often discouraged to use products that contain THC. There may be some benefits that come from marijuana consumption, but the negatives that come from THC often outweigh those. But this is where CBD oil comes in. It provides you with all of the benefits that you are looking for, without worrying about any of the negative effects that we have just stated.

The science behind CBD oil and how it helps heal the body

Before you make the decision to use CBD oil, it is important to learn as much about cannabidiol as possible. This is the main ingredient in these oils and will provide you with all of the benefits that you are hoping to gain in the process. But how does all of this work?

CBD, or the cannabidiol, is going to be the main compound that is found in hemp. Unlike what we see with THC, it is not going to be psychoactive, so you won't have to worry about being high. Cannabidiol works because it interacts with your CB receptors through the endocannabinoid system in order to provide you with all of the good benefits that you hear about with this kind of oil.

First, we need to take a look at the two receptors that make this possible. The cannabinoid receptors are going to be the main players for a series of processes that occur in the human body. This can include regulating your memory, your appetite, pain sensation, and your mood.

These receptors are sometimes activated by the endocannabinoids, which are the chemicals that are produced in the human body. But they can also be activated by cannabinoids that come from plants as well, including those found in cannabis and hemp. There are many receptors in the body, but they are grouped into two categories, mainly the CB1 and CB2 receptors.

To start are the CB1 receptors. These are the ones that are found in the central nervous system, although it is possible to find them in the lungs, kidneys, and liver, even though they are there in smaller amounts. When we look for the CB2 receptors, they are part of your immune system. CB1 receptors are the ones that are responsible for the production and release of neurotransmitters, which is when the cannabis products that affect these can often lead to feeling high or other negative side effects.

You will also find that these CB1 receptors are involved in what is known as the lipogenesis process, which is going to take place in the liver. It can also play a major role in the maintenance of homeostasis, which is the equilibrium that the body tries to stick with. While there needs to be more studies done on this, it is suggested that CB1 may also be able to influence pain tolerance, memory, appetite, concentration, and also pleasure.

Then there are the CB2 receptors. These are going to be the receptors that work closely with the immune system. They involve themselves in many different functions such as apoptosis, or programmed death of the cells, and immune suppression. Studies often suggest that these CB2 receptors are going to modulate the sensation of pain and may be able to help prevent or lessen the effects of many serious diseases.

The activation of the adenosine receptors, like what is done when you take in CBD oil, can provide you with a lot of nutritive benefits. These can help the body fight off issues such as with inflammation and anxiety. These same receptors are going to also helps to release glutamate and dopamine, which are both going to help with motor control, memory, learning, cognition, and even the reward mechanisms.

When all of these come together, it is easy to see how CBD oil is able to help with so many different disorders and issues in the body. It has the ability to inhibit and activate the right receptors so that the body can act in the way that it should. This results in less anxiety, a limited amount of inflammation, help with depression, diabetes, heart health, and so much more.

How is CBD different from marijuana?

To someone who hasn't had a chance to look at these two products, it may seem like hemp and marijuana are similar. But if you already have an idea of what to look for, you will be able to see some distinctions. To start, hemp and marijuana are actually species of cannabis and they both come from the Cannabis Sativa family. Since they come from the same family, there are going to be some similarities. But since they are both different biologically, there are some very crucial differences.

Hemp CBD, which is the one that we are going to talk about in this guidebook, is going to be very high in CBD and low on THC. This means that you are able to get an oil that is high on cannabidiol and other essential fatty acids, minerals, and vitamins to help keep the body healthy and get it to function properly, without having any of the negative THC which will cause you to get high.

It is possible to grow hemp with some cross-pollination in order to get the higher levels of CBD that are needed. However, the original hemp plant just doesn't have the amount of CBD that is needed to provide the medicinal effects that the user is looking for. This means that different strains (like some of the ones that we will talk about later on), have to be developed in order to get the right levels of CBD and the right levels of THC to get the full effects.

Marijuana, on the other hand, is going to have higher levels of the THC that we talked about before. While there may be some CBD that is found in it, you will find that this is not the primary thing that growers of marijuana are looking for. In fact, most suppliers of marijuana aim to get the THC content as high as possible to beat out the competition.

With marijuana, the majority of users are not going to focus on using it to improve their health. Instead, they use it as a way to help them get high or experience a number of other psychoactive effects in the body. They may use it to help them relax and mellow out, but they want to do so while getting high, rather than doing it as a way to just naturally heal the body. The THC levels of CBD oil must be below 0.3 percent, but the THC levels in marijuana are going to be much higher.

Marijuana is going to provide the body with a high, which is preferable to some users. But it can cause a ton of negative health effects and you need to be careful about the dosage that you take. With CBD oil, you don't have to worry about the dosage being too high because it is considered safe for most people. This makes the CBD oil a much better option when you actually want to improve your overall health.

Is it safe for me to use?

CBD oil is safe for you to use. While there may be a few side effects, mostly from taking a substandard version of the product, most people are able to take this oil without any issues at all. Since these oils are non-psychoactive and have minimal side effects, this can be one of the best ways for you to improve your health with minimal side effects.

There are several benefits that come with taking this oil, and these ensure that the oil is safe for you and other members of your family to use. CBD has been tested as safe, as well as non-toxic, for humans, even when it is taken in higher amounts. According to research that was developed by the University of Sao Paulo Brazil, CBD is safe and non-toxic in both animals and humans. In fact, this same research team stated that even really high doses, up to 1500 mg each day of this oil could still be tolerated well in humans.

Of course, most individuals won't need that much oil during the day. Most people will be fine taking 300 mg or less for the entire day. If you are safe at 1500, then the 300 won't bother you or cause any toxic effects on your body.

In addition, CBD oil is considered non-psychoactive. While marijuana has been bred to contain higher levels of THC to help create the euphoric effects that people purchase it for, hemp is going to contain lower levels of his chemical. In fact, for cannabis to be considered hemp at all, it must be at 0.3 percent or lower of THC per dry weight. Instead of holding onto the higher levels of THC, it contains more cannabidiol/CBD.

The CBD isn't going to cause you to get high like THC does. Instead, it interacts with the receptors of the body and helps to maintain the natural balance that is found in the body. THC is going to work with the CB1 receptors in order to generate a psychoactive effect, but CBD will work with the CB2 receptor in order to help promote a number of health benefits in the body. Since there are only trace amounts of the THC inside these mixtures, it is safe for you to use without any negative side effects.

To add to all of this, there aren't any major side effects that come with using this substance. You may experience dry mouth, some drowsiness or the opposite effect of wakefulness, and some lower blood pressure issues. But compared to some of the medications that the CBD oil will replace, the side effects are minimal and you will love how much better you feel in no time.

Are there any effects of using CBD and hemp oil?

There are so many great health benefits that come with using CBD oil in your own life. And since the research into this is growing so much, it is likely that even more great benefits and effects that come with using it. There is almost nothing that can't be cured and helped when it comes to taking CBD oil, you just have to figure out the right dosage for the condition that you want to work on.

Some of the effects of using CBD oil that are already recognized and established, and even have had some research done on them include:

1. Can relieve pain, including muscle pain, headaches, and arthritis.
2. Can help you to reduce depression and anxiety that you may feel.

3. Has the ability to alleviate cancer-related symptoms and may be able to stop cancer.
4. Could help to reduce acne.
5. Can help protect the brain and prevent many neurological conditions.
6. Can help benefit the health of your heart. It can do this by reducing your blood pressure, preventing diabetes, reducing the stress that you feel, and so much more.
7. Can help as a treatment for many mental disorders by reducing the number of psychotic symptoms the patient has.
8. CBD can also help to change up the circuits in the brain when it comes to addiction to drugs. In fact, in some studies of rats, this chemical has been shown to reduce morphine dependence as well as behavior for seeking heroin.
9. Can help prevent diabetes. In mice who suffered from diabetes, treatment with CBD was able to reduce the incidences of diabetes by about 56 percent. There was

also a significant reduction in inflammation through the body.

How long does it take to feel the effects?

There are a number of factors that come into play when determining how long it will take for the CBD oil to work. It can vary between a few minutes to a few hours or more before you see relief, so make sure that you give yourself some time. Depending on the dosage that you take, the method of consumption, and what symptoms you are looking to alleviate, the time is going to vary.

If you are vaping or taking in the CBD sublingually, you may be able to feel the effects of this chemical in just a few minutes. This is part of why these versions are the preferred ones to go with. Sufferers don't want to wait around all day to feel some relief and see if the oil works. But if you choose to have an edible form of CBD, such as adding the oil into some desserts, then it may take a few hours before you feel it kick in.

The preferred method for taking in the CBD oil is to either vape or take it in your mouth through oral drops where it will be absorbed there. This gets them right over to the receptors that you want in no time at all. You can also try applying these products topically, but again, you have to wait for them to absorb in the body, and this can take some time.

Some patients like to have edibles with the oil inside it. They like the taste and find that they can handle the oil a bit easier when they do this method. But any time that you add the oil into some food or you combine it with any type of food or drink, you may have to wait a bit longer for the results. But the good news is that the taste is often better and you won't have to worry about the side effects because you ensure that there is something in your stomach at the time.

The amount of time that is considered for the effects of CBD oil to take place is going to depend on these factors and more. If you take in a larger dose, you will feel it faster. If you decide to vape the oil or take it sublingually, you will notice that it hits you faster. But if you take a smaller dosage or you decide to take it in an edible form or topically, it may take a bit longer to feel the results.

How long do the effects last?

The CBD oil can often last in your system for several days, which can provide you relief from some of your serious symptoms for a good amount of time. There are several things that will influence how long the effects last in your body though. For example, your metabolism is going to play a big role in how long it will take the body to process this oil. If your metabolism is faster, then you may find that the oil doesn't last as long as it does for others. Generally, the oil is able to remain in your system, at least in trace amounts, for about three days or more.

The potency of the oil, and how much you take in can greatly affect how long the oil lasts. If you only take a small dosage, like 2 or 3mg, then you will find that the effects may not last long and you will often need to take more dosages. But if you take 300mg, it may last you all day before you need to go through another dosage.

Depending on the mode of use when it comes to the oil, the effects of CBD oil can last somewhere between two to six hours. The topicals will often last the longest because it takes them a bit longer to absorb. This is then followed by the capsules and the edibles. This means that you may need to take a few dosages of the medication or treatment to ensure the effects can help with your condition through the whole day.

Chapter 2

How CBD Can Help Alleviate Your Aches and Pains

For most of us, a little bit of pain on occasion is not a big deal. We may have to take some medication to help out if it gets really bad, but overall we feel just fine and can go about our normal day. But for some people, those aches and pains can start to take over. The pain can make even regular and everyday activities seem almost impossible to keep up with. They may have tried different activities, exercises, and medications, but the pain can come in and make it very hard to even function and do the things that you really want to do.

CBD Oil is a great alternative that you may want to consider when your chronic pain is making things especially difficult. This oil has been proven to work on relieving a lot of different types of chronic pain.

Even individuals who have tried everything, and been in pain for years, found that CBD oil could help them reduce and even eliminate the amount of pain that they felt. Even better is the fact that CBD provides this relief without the harmful side effects that come with traditional pain medications.

While the legal status of CBD oil is still uncertain in many parts of the country, there is a legal provision that will allow patients to use medical marijuana to help them deal with this chronic pain, as long as it is used with the permission of your doctor. There are a few other requirements that need to be met to get this oil in prescription, but it can still help to bring this in the right direction.

Even though there is some limitation on getting ahold of medical marijuana to treat this kind of chronic pain, CBD can still be a great oil to use in order to help you get healthier and get rid of the chronic pain that you are dealing with. And as the population of our country starts to age more, it is likely that the problem with chronic pain is going to continue to grow and more and more people will want to start using CBD oil to reduce pain.

So at this point, you may be wondering if CBD really is effective when it comes to reducing chronic pain and can it get the job done?

A study was done in 2008 to check and see the efficacy of cannabinoids, outside of how effective THC is when it comes to pain management.

In this study, it showed that the participants were able to handle painkillers with cannabinoids in them, and there were minimum side effects in the process. There also weren't any issues with toxicity in the body from taking these kinds of painkillers. When the CBD was combined together with opioids, the effect was even more pronounced, showing that this may be the future that we are looking for when it comes to taking care of chronic pain.

How can CBD oil help reduce inflammation

Inflammation has always been a little bit tricky to deal with when it comes to finding good solutions to help with it. The most promising area that has been studied so far has taken a look at the endocannabinoid system, namely both the CB1 and CB2 receptor activation.

The cannabidiol that is found in CBD is going to react with this system in a very interesting way. In fact, it appears that this reaction could be promising when it comes to how CBD can help reduce inflammation, especially for those who have been dealing with inflammation in the body. This could mean relief for millions of people who are suffering from pain and a host of other health issues related to inflammation.

There has been a lot of interest in research to look into how Cannabidiol can work to help prevent pain and prevent inflammation in the body. Traditional painkillers and other treatments may help in some cases, but often they don't treat the root of the inflammation. So, even if it does provide you with some relief from the pain that you feel, it is likely that you are still experiencing the inflammation and it is still causing some damage.

While other methods may not provide relief or cessation to inflammation, there have been many positive findings when it comes to studying the endocannabinoid system. These studies are going to focus on what happens when the CB1 and CB2 receptors and how they are affected by both CBD and HC.

CBD can work as an anti-inflammatory agent by activating these receptors. Remember that inflammation is a response from the immune system, which CB2 controls. But when the CBD oil meets with these receptors, it can help to calm and control the inflammation.

The great news here is that not only does the CBD help to reduce the inflammation by calming down the immune system, but it also helps out with other immune system problems, or at least other illnesses and conditions that are in part linked back to the immune system. This can include a lot of different health conditions including hypertension, atherosclerosis, arthritis, depression, metabolic syndrome, Alzheimer's disease, both types of diabetes, and much more.

Even better, the research that has looked into this shows that while CBD oil is able to help deal with inflammation, there are very few side effects to using this treatment. Since the oil doesn't have THC or very low concentrations of it, the CB1 receptors will not be affected at all. This results in absolutely no psychoactive effects that come with consuming cannabis. All that you will see with this kind of oil is the benefits, and an overall feeling better in the body. It is natural, effective, and can help you to fight off inflammation through the body while having fewer bad side effects in the process.

Chapter 3

DEPRESSION AND ANXIETY

Depression and anxiety are two of the most common issues that many people suffer with. While having a down mood or feeling a bit anxious on occasion is completely normal, there are times when this can be taken to the next level, and these conditions can start to take over your life. It is possible to use CBD oil to help alleviate these issues making you feel better.

Using CBD oil to help with depression

According to the American Psychiatric Association, the disorder of depression is affecting about one in fifteen adults every year, and almost one in six people will experience depression at one point or another in their lives. For anyone who suffers from depression, or if you know someone who deals with depression, it is easy to agree that this is a disorder that can really debilitate the individual and can make life hard to deal with.

The good news is that you may be able to use CBD to help handle and improve your depression for the better. CBD is actually one of the 60+ naturally occurring compounds that you are able to find in the cannabis plant. When we look at the human body, there are endocannabinoids that will be the chemical messengers to a special part of the nervous system. The endocannabinoid system is the part that will contain cannabinoid cell receptors that are able to respond to the cannabinoids, such as those found in CBD, which tells the body to do different things.

The human body is actually able to produce some of its own cannabinoids with the help of some fatty acids (you can consume these fatty acids in a variety of foods like fish, seeds, and nuts). These same receptors are going to be able to form a bond with the compounds that are found in cannabis.

Unlike what we find with THC, CBD has a different, and somewhat more indirect, interaction when it comes to these specific cell receptors. At the same time, it is possible for the CBD to interact with the other receptors, including the receptors for dopamine and serotonin. Because of this, when you ingest some CBD oil, it is able to influence the brain. One of the byproducts that you see from this is that dopamine and serotonin are released through the body.

There have been two recent studies that help to uncover how CBD oil is able to help in dealing with the symptoms that come with depression. In one of these studies, which was done in 2011, researchers spent some time looking at the modulation of the serotonin system through signaling of the endocannabinoid. In this research, they found that there was plenty of evidence to show that these endocannabinoids were going to be regulators when it came to stress responses. What this means is that there can be the assumption that during depression, taking in CBD may be able to help the individual regulate how they respond to situations they find stressful.

In addition, researchers from the University of San Paulo in Brazil, along with researchers at King's

College in London, found that, when there were high enough concentrations of the CBD, it was able to directly activate the receptor for serotonin. What this did in the body was help provide a type of anti-anxiety effect on the body.

While there have been a lot of independent studies and even testimonials that give those suffering from this depression some hope for a natural alternative to help them deal with their depression, there needs to be some more research done to make sure that this is a safe and effective method to help you deal with your depression. If you are looking to help yourself deal with a down mood on occasion, then it may be a good idea to try CBD oil. But if you are already on medications, make sure to discuss this with your doctor before dropping the medication altogether.

How can CBD help with Anxiety?

Another condition that a lot of people deal with on a regular basis is anxiety. Anxiety can sometimes occur along with depression and other times it is going to occur on its own. Depending on how severe the anxiety is, it could take over the life of the sufferer. It can feel like a weight that can keep them back from the things that they want to get done. They may avoid certain situations and people in order to avoid feeling the panic attacks that can come with anxiety.

It is normal to have a bit of anxiety on occasion. When we have to get up and talk in front of other people, when we have to go in for an interview, or when we are taking a big important test. All of these can lead us to feel anxious and like we want to just go back home. It is normal to feel anxiety on these occasions. But the anxiety that we are talking about is the one that shows up all of the time. It is the anxiety that is going to make it difficult to do even normal things during the day. And it can turn you into someone you may not recognize. If the anxiety gets bad enough, it is possible that the individual will avoid situations, change their job, refuse to go out, and even do other things in their lives to make sure that they don't end up in a situation where they will start to have anxiety.

Since problems with anxiety have the ability to change up almost every aspect of your life if you let it, it is very important for these individuals to look for a cure, one that is going to help them manage their anxiety, and allows them to get their lives back on track. They know that the anxiety is not supposed to be there. They know that their fears are taking over their lives and that it is not reasonable for you to feel that way.

The traditional methods of working with anxiety are not that effective at dealing with the problem. They often come with a ton of side effects that are worse than the anxiety itself, and many of them don't do anything for the side effects at all. They may also try to do some form of therapy, this can sometimes work but not always, as the therapist must have the right training to deal with this issue in specific.

The good news here is that the CBD oil is a viable cure that has had some success. The anxiolytic effect of THC is documented in many different studies and when it is combined with other cannabinoids, such as CBD, it is also able to provide relief to the user. The exact way that this works in the body is not yet certain. However, a preliminary study that was published in 2013 in the International

Neuropsychopharmacology Journal has set the foundation for more research in the future to show that CBD could be a great treatment for anxiety and for depression in many patients.

This is great news for those who are suffering from severe anxiety that is influencing their lives. This is especially true for those who are dealing with anxiety that has not been cured by other options. CBD oil is very effective at helping to calm the individual down and helping them to feel less excitement or worry. And without all the bad side effects that come with some other anxiety medications that are in the market, it is certainly something that should be looked into in the future.

Chapter 4

Other Health Benefits

In addition to some of the benefits we discussed in previous chapters, there are many other reasons why people will choose to add CBD oil into their lives. Knowing that there isn't enough THC in the mixture to cause them to get high can help to open up a world of opportunities and better health for almost anyone.

Many of those who start looking into the benefits of CBD oil will do so because they are tired of all the bad health they currently have in their lives. And in many cases, they may have already tried many other methods to improve their health, without any success. They may have talked to their doctor, tried to change their diet, went on countless medications and treatments, and yet they still suffer. Then they hear about CBD oil and decide to investigate whether it could be the cure they are looking for.

Of course, not everyone who comes to CBD oil has a major health issue that they are trying to solve. Some just want to feel better, have more energy, or deal with a smaller health concern that they want to see improve. What this means is that there are a lot of different reasons and a lot of different kinds of people who will try out CBD oil to help them get to feeling better.

Before we get a look at some of the other health concerns that CBD can help with, we need to remember that just like any other medication, CBD oil is going to work differently in each person. You may find that you need a slightly higher dose than someone else, or maybe you need a little less. Maybe this oil can make one condition better for you but doesn't seem to work as well in another condition. This is why experimenting a bit with the dosage and the type of oil you go with can be so important to get the most out of this treatment.

Even though it may take a bit of time to get the right dosage of CBD oil for your health needs, this treatment is still effective for a wide variety of diseases and illnesses. In fact, many claim that CBD can be more effective than the medication they receive from a pharmacy. Let's take a look at some of the different health benefits you can get when you use CBD oil.

Cancer and chemotherapy

One health benefit that is getting a lot of attention is how CBD oil can help with cancer and can lessen the negative side effects that come during the chemotherapy treatment. CBD oil is full of many anti-emetic and anti-nausea chemicals, which can help patients feel better, and even keep their appetites up when they undergo chemotherapy. About twenty years ago, these two factors of CBD were attributed to the actions of the THC chemical. Over time, further research into these cannabinoids showed that there are actually a ton of different chemicals that are inside cannabis that can produce the same effects as THC in cancer patients, but without having to introduce the negative side effects that come with THC.

In fact, CBD oil has become such a powerful treatment for chemotherapy patients that the FDA already recommends the use of two mainstream drugs that feature these cannabinoids in them. And out of the two, CBD oil has the highest concentration of those chemicals.

How can you use this to help with chemotherapy? When you are undergoing this treatment, taking CBD oil can help to reduce the amount and severity of nausea that patients may feel during and afterward. For many patients, this can be the answer they are looking for to help them feel better, to increase appetite so they can heal, and to increase the outlook of their cancer prognosis.

In addition, there are some newer studies that suggest that CBD oil should be incorporated into various cancer therapies to make them more efficient. Adding this in as a regular part of cancer treatments such as chemotherapy could make it easier for patients to get back to normal once they are done.

In addition, specialists at the National Cancer Institute have found that CBD oil could be used in other ways as well when it comes to cancer. These specialists took some time to review experiments that have been done on rodents and rhesus monkeys. The results of this review implied that CBD may be able to inhibit the division that we see in cancerous cells, and this is even more apparent in certain cancers like leukemia and lymphoma. These same chemicals could also lower the probability that the tissues that were already affected would then start to spread over to other parts of the body.

This is good news on several levels. Not only could the chemicals in CBD help patients who are undergoing chemotherapy by helping them to avoid nausea and the other harmful side effects, but these chemicals could also be used in a way to help prevent the spread of cancer, making chemotherapy more efficient and preventing more complications around the way.

This is great news for those who are dealing with cancer on several levels. The first one is that if you are dealing with cancer and undergoing chemotherapy, it is possible to take the CBD oil in order to help with the nausea that is experienced. Many people who have gone through cancer or who have seen loved ones go through cancer understand that the nausea and the issues of not being able to eat during the treatment can be hard on anyone. The use of CBD oil can help to reduce the nausea in patients so that they can have a better experience while dealing with cancer.

As if all of that weren't enough, it is possible that CBD oil could also be used as a treatment by itself, instead of putting the patient through chemotherapy at all. Some patients in beginning studies have taken this oil and seen that it has helped them in improving their cancer. This works because the oil is going to inhibit cancer cells from dividing and growing, and since the oil can prevent these cancerous cells from moving around the body, there is less risk of the cancer spreading.

Even though a lot of the research into CBD oil and cancer is relatively new, this is still promising news for those who are dealing with cancer or who have a loved one who has dealt with cancer in the past or present. This may be just the solution that we have been waiting for to fight off this horrible disease and keep it away, without all the invasive treatments.

Diabetes and heart disease

As we discussed before, CBD oil will come with a wide range of anti-inflammatory properties. Because of this, the oil is able to help with many heart conditions, and with diabetes. CBD can be effective for a number of reasons in helping treat both of these common ailments. But the biggest reason is that of the reduction of inflammation throughout the body leads to a reduction in insulin resistance and an increase in insulin sensitivity. This leads to fewer sugars hanging around the body and can help the heart work more efficiently.

Since the 1990s when CBD was first discovered, there has been some who speculate that it was able to have a good effect on more than just the cannabinoid receptors of the body, that it could have an effect on other types of receptors as well. If this were true, it stands to reason that this chemical could be used in treatments to help with a variety of heart conditions such as atherosclerosis.

This has lead to several studies done on this issue. In fact, researchers from the University of Tel Aviv took the time to finish studies that showed that when giving CBD to rodents who had areas of dead tissue in their heart muscle, there was a 30 percent increase in blood flow afterward. This could be great news for patients who are already suffering from heart conditions or those who are candidates for these issues and who want to stop it before things get worse.

Muscle spasms and seizures

CBD oil has always had kind of a murky relationship with the law. While it technically doesn't contain THC in it and won't get the user high, there are some states and areas that still won't allow it. And even with those that do, there is a fine line between what is legal and what isn't. But one of the main reasons that people are easily able to get their hands on this oil legally, is to help with muscle spasms such as seizures.

There have been many cases where children, as well as adults, who suffer from what is known as extreme seizure disorders. Often these conditions were so bad that the individuals had an almost impossible time living their lives. They tried many different treatments, and none of them were providing these individuals with any sort of relief. For those who started taking a treatment of CBD oil, it was found that the seizures either stopped completely, or they were reduced to such a number that the individual was able to begin leading a normal life again. Because of these studies, it is believed that CBD oil is an effective and natural cure that can help sufferers of severe seizures, as well as other conditions, without causing negative side effects.

The information that was shown in the above section was meant to relate chiefly to epilepsy, and the FDA currently allows epilepsy centers throughout the United States to prescribe products that contain CBD in them to patients, as long as these patients are not responding to classical medication.

The reason that this is now allowed for some patients is that of a comprehensive study that was done in 2015 and was aimed at two very difficult forms of epilepsy known as Lennox-Gastaut syndrome and Dravet syndrome. These two forms are most often experienced in children and because of this, it is sometimes hard to find the right dosage and the right types of medications to help with the disorders.

However, these children were able to use CBD oil in order to help them reduce their seizure frequency and could help them to almost disappear in some situations. For example, those who took cannabidiol medication for six months found a decrease between 54 and 67 percent during that time. It is important to note that the CBD oil is effective, but it does not work in every patient. There were some in the study above who stopped taking the CBD oil after three months because it did not help their conditions improve at all.

Autoimmune disorders

Another way that you can use your CBD oil is to deal with autoimmune disorders. Most of these are going to be caused by the inflammation that occurs in your body. There are a variety of reasons that you may have this inflammation present, but the big issue is that it can seriously make you sick. Using CBD oil may be able to reduce the inflammation in the body, the same inflammation that is known for causing arthritis and joint pain.

If you are looking to reduce the amount of inflammation that is in the body so you can fight off diabetes, heart conditions, arthritis, and other joint pain, then it may be best to try out some CBD oil. There are a lot of painkillers and pain relief options that are out on the market, but none of them are most likely not to be as effective as working with CBD oil.

Fibromyalgia

Some sufferers of fibromyalgia have reported relief from their pain when taking medical marijuana and CBD oil to help with the symptoms. In fact, many of them claim that these products are more effective at helping out with these symptoms than the prescription medications they were on before. According to numbers given out by the National Institutes of Health, it is estimated that at least 5 million Americans suffer from this condition, which means they are suffering from symptoms like headaches, depression, hard time sleeping, deep tissue pain, and fatigue.

Respondents to a survey done by the National Institutes of Health claim that they have tried one or more medications to help with their symptoms, but many of these same respondents tried all three major medications that are FDA approved. At least 60 percent said that these medications provided them with no relief and claimed that the negative side effects from taking the medication really weren't worth the relief they got.

However, when the respondents tried cannabis and CBD oil to help with the symptoms of fibromyalgia, 62 percent said that it was effective at relieving their symptoms with few side effects, and another 33 percent on top of that said the product helps them at least a little. This means that only 5 percent of the respondents who tried cannabis and CBD oil didn't receive any relief, compared to the up to 70 percent on traditional medications.

Post-traumatic stress disorder

Some sufferers of PTSD found that CBD was effective at treating the symptoms they had. The biggest issue here is that most of those who suffer from this disorder choose to self-medicate, so finding the right research and information is more difficult compared to the other disorders.

PSD is a disorder that makes it hard for the individual to cope with daily life. They may have troubles dealing with intrusive memories and thoughts, have sleep problems, hyperarousal and nightmares on a regular basis. These can get so bad that they disrupt the normal day to day functioning of the individual.

Taking a bit of CBD oil on a daily basis has proven to be a great way to get relief from these symptoms. Many individuals with PTSD claim that this oil has helped them to limit or eliminate their anxiety and it helps them to relax. While the patient still needs to seek counseling and other methods to help deal with the root of the PTSD, these oils can help to relax the patient and can make them more receptive to the effects of the other treatments.

Can be used to help with weight loss

There are some people who are looking into this oil, and other similar treatments, to help with weight loss. The studies that have been done on this took a look at how CBD oil can be a great appetite suppressant. The conclusion is that by consuming CBD oil you will get the following effects:

1. The oil was able to help reduce the expression of protein that is involved in lipogenesis or fat cell production.
2. The oil was able to increase the number and the activity of the mitochondria, which is needed to help burn calories faster than before.
3. This oil is able to stimulate the genes and the proteins in the body. This helps to encourage the breakdown and the oxidation of fats in the body to encourage weight loss.

If you have been struggling to lose weight and have tried all of the other tricks and cures, then it may be time to try out CBD oil. It may be just what you need to burn off more fat, suppress the appetite, and speed up your metabolism.

If you are enjoying the audiobook, I would love if you went to Audible and left a short review.

Chapter 5

The Essentials to Know When Buying CBD Oils

Sometimes the hardest part of this process is finding high-quality products to use. There aren't many regulations on CBD oil, which means that the strains, the concentrations, and the product that you get will be different depending on the supplier you work with. While there are many reputable suppliers you can purchase from, there are also a lot of suppliers who just want to jump on board and will sell products that are not effective, and some that aren't even that safe to consume.

Making smart decisions and being an intelligent consumer can go a long way in helping you to get the right kinds of CBD oil for your needs. Let's take a look at some of the different factors that you must consider when you are ready to purchase CBD oil for yourself.

How do I know when I am getting a product that is high quality?

If you want to get the effects of CBD oil, then you must make sure that you are purchasing high-quality products. There are many different suppliers on the market, and since there isn't any regulation on them, it is hard to get the same quality in products from different sellers.

Of course, a lot of these suppliers make this their income, and they will strive hard to give you a high-quality oil that you will love. But then there are also those who just want to get in the market to make money quickly, and often sell low quality products. The good news is that even though there are no regulations out there right now when it comes to CBD oil, there are a few key factors that you can look for to ensure you get the best quality product possible.

The first thing you should look at is the source of the oil. You will need to see where the oil and plant comes from before it is processed. Often you are going to see that the hemp comes from China. This is a popular option because this often costs less so suppliers can offer a good product for less money and still turn a profit. However, this isn't always the highest quality hemp. It is fine and won't be a bad thing if you use it, but if you want the highest quality product, then try to look for oils that have their hemp sourced from Europe, the United States, or Australia. This leads to a higher price on the product, but will be worth it in terms of quality.

The next thing that you should look at is the petroleum-free processing. The way that your suppliers takes the CBD from the plant can be very important. The best method is known as a chemical-free cold CO_2 extraction because it helps the producer and supplier get the most CBD out of the plant as possible. This method can be more expensive than others, which is why you may see some producers choose to go with a different method.

Even though there are other methods, it is best to choose suppliers who use the chemical-free cold CO_2 extraction method. The solvents that are used in this method are safer and they can ensure that you end up with an extract that is pure and very potent. Other benefits of this method include it being eco-friendly, non-toxic, and its effect on the environment is minimal.

Always make sure that you check out whether or not the supplier has independent lab results to go with the product. For some of the smaller suppliers, you aren't going to get this because they don't have the resources to make it happen. But if it is a bigger company, make sure to check all of these out. Finding a company that can offer these lab results can give a bit of reassurance that the oil is safe, and can ensure that the oil is higher in quality.

One of the benefits of working with CBD and hemp oil rather than marijuana is that it has a low level of THC in it. This allows the individual to get the benefits they want out of the oil, without having to worry about getting high or suffering from any other negative side effects. When you are searching for oils, you must make sure that the levels of THC are kept to a minimum.

The best CBD oil is going to come with levels of THC that are below .03 percent. The lower you can get this amount, the better. The point of this is to make sure that you get lots of good benefits from the CBD that is in the oil, without the bad effects that comes with the THC. There are a few options you can choose that have a higher THC content, and they will probably be fine to consume.

Finally, make sure that you find an oil that uses the whole plant. This means that the oil you get is going to be taken from all of the plants, and that includes the stem, the stalks, and the seeds of the plant. This helps you to get more than just the CBD; you will also get the other natural chemicals that come in the plant such as the sugars, flavonoids, terpenes, and secondary cannabinoids. All of these chemicals can come together to increase how effective CBD can be for the body.

There are some suppliers who focus on just adding the CBD alone into the oil and will just try to sell it like that. But if you want the best quality, and the one that will provide you with the most health benefits, then you should find one that has the whole plant in it as well.

What concentration of CBD should be in the product?

Just like with other products you may use, CBD can be watered down in some products. It is possible that some companies will try to gain more profits by diluting the oil and then tricking their customers into thinking they are getting more for less, even though they aren't getting the concentration they think they are. It is very important for you to pay attention to the concentration of the oil you are buying, to ensure you get the strength and quality you are looking for.

There is a wide range of concentrations that you will find. But most products are going to have somewhere between 250 and 1000mg per fluid ounce of the CBD. This is going to matter quite a bit in reality. If you purchased a bottle that was four ounces and it contained just 250mg of CBD, the concentration would only be 62.5mg per ounce. This isn't very much at all, and you probably won't really benefit from it.

If you find that the concentration of the CBD isn't on the bottle, then there is a formula that you can use to help you figure this out on your own. This would be taking the total amount of CBD and divide by the volume that is found in the container. An example of this would be:

1500mg/ 4 ounce bottle = 375mg/oz.

How do I know that the oil is pure and potent?

Always look for the Lab reports on a potential brand of CBD oil you are looking at buying. A third-party accredited laboratory will be used to test the potency of the oil and is the best and only way to guarantee the oils quality, and safety of use.

The accredited laboratory should take the time to test a bunch of things in the oil including:

- ❖ If there are heavy metals inside it
- ❖ Foreign matter

- Microbes
- Bacteria and fungus
- Any residual chemical solvents that come from the process of extraction
- Pesticides

How much should I spend on the product?

While everyone would love to get a good deal on the product that they have, remember that in this case, cheaper is not always better. In many cases, cheaper means that the production quality of the CBD isn't cheap and if someone offers a price that is too low, then there is a higher likelihood of toxic solvents and other residue left in the product. This oil is definitely something that you should spend a little extra to make sure that you get a good product.

While the CO_2 extraction is going to get you a higher price tag when you purchase the product, it will ensure that it has a good potency, purity, and quality, especially when used to extract CBD oil from the hemp product organically grown in the United States. There are a few different reasons that you may find that an oil is priced a bit higher and these include:

- ❖ It is made from an extract that is full spectrum and high quality. This ensures that some other compounds that can be beneficial for your health are present.
- ❖ The company is following the laws and the rules of that area.
- ❖ The product has been tested in a third party lab.
- ❖ The product is grown in the United States.
- ❖ There is a higher concentration of CBD in the product.
- ❖ The CBD was extracted with the help of the CO_2 method
- ❖ The product was grown organically.

How do I find a good supplier?

Once you know what to look for in your product, it is easier than ever to find a good supplier. You first need to find someone who has a product that includes all of the things that we discussed previously, and you already have a good start. The first thing to consider is the type of product they provide, and the method you will need to use to take it. Do you want to take a pill, a few drops, a spray, or a concentrate? This can help limit some of your potential choices. There are some suppliers that will offer a few different choices, but then there are some that just offer one option.

The price of the product is important. After searching through a few suppliers, you should be able to tell what the average price is per ounce for each type of oil. While everyone wants to get a good deal on the product they get, you also have to be careful because if the product is priced way too low, then it could mean you aren't getting a high-quality product. These suppliers may add extra stuff to the product or they may dilute the oil until it isn't useful. Compare prices to help you find an oil that has everything you need and comes in at an affordable price.

Depending on the area you live in, you may only be able to find a supplier online because none are in your area. There are many reputable sellers online you can choose from. Make sure to read through the reviews on each seller to see what other customers thought and if there were any problems with a particular seller or not.

Chapter 6

Consumption

Now that we know a little bit more about CBD oil and all of the great benefits that come with it, it is time to move on to actually consuming the oil. You can't get the benefits of this oil without first consuming the oil for yourself. The good news is, this process is relatively simple and there are a few different methods that you can choose from to fit your needs. Let's dive into some of the different methods for consuming CBD oil, along with the other factors that you should consider to get started.

Different methods of consuming CBD oil

There are actually a few different methods that you can use in order to take in the CBD oil that you want to consume. The method that you decide to go with will be up to personal preference, and can sometimes vary based on the reason that you are using the oil. Some of the different methods that you can choose from when you want to consume the CBD oil include:

Tinctures:

This is the most common way that the oil is applied. This is often the purest application of the oil because there won't be any processing done on the oil to make it in the right form. It is possible to get a bit of flavoring to the oil if you don't like the original. The flavoring can make it easier for you to consume the oil, but it is not necessary to add this in.

To do a tincture, you simply need to add a few drops, either under or on the tongue depending on your preference. We will talk about the dosage in a bit, but most of them are going to range between 100mg and 1000mg for the tincture. If this is your first time, start out with the 100mg and build up to where you need it. The biggest issue you may encounter with the tincture is it can make a bit of a mess, and some people don't like the taste of it. You can always add in the flavoring to help though.

The most effective way to take the tincture is to not swallow the liquid the moment it touches your tongue. Instead, try placing a few drops on the cheek or right under the tongue and then leave them there to absorb for a few minutes or aslong as the instructions on the bottle tell you to. If you do swallow a bit, that is not a big deal, but giving the tincture some time to absorb can really make a difference.

Concentrates

If you are looking for a method to use that has the strongest amount of CBD in it, then the concentrates are the right one for you. With that said, make sure to read the dosage properly because these can have ten times or more the concentrate of the other options, and you don't want to overdo it and take in too much. Some patients choose to go with the concentrate instead of a tincture because it is faster and more convenient to use.

The biggest issue that comes with the concentrate is its lack of flavor. This usually isn't a big deal, but some people find that the natural flavor of the oil can be really bad tasting and hard to swallow. This becomes even worse because the CBD is found in such high concentrations in these products. You may want to try a sample of this first and see if it is really the right option for you.

Many customers like to go with the concentrates because they are higher potency so you can get the right dosage without it taking a long time. To use this version of the oil, you just need to place it along the cheek or under the tongue and then give it some time to dissolve.

Capsules

The next option on the list is capsules. This is the easiest method to use because you would take it just like you would take a daily multivitamin. Many customers find that this is an easy method to use and if you already take a supplement for some other reason, you can easily add in the CBD capsules to your daily regimen to get some results as well.

When you take the capsules, you are going to get a little lower concentration of the CBD compared to some other methods. These usually come in around 10 to 25 mg of CBD. And since they come in predetermined amounts of oil to start with, it is easier to control your dosage, rather than hoping you measured it out correctly. They do make it a bit harder to experiment with your dosage since they are in set amounts, but for most people, this isn't a big deal. To take the capsules, you just take the dose you need with some water each day.

Topicals

There are now a lot of different topicals out there, like lotions, lip balms, and more, that contain this oil in them due to some of the great skin benefits. These topicals can help with a bunch of different things like psoriasis, acne, anti-aging, inflammation, and sometimes it is used in a topical form to help with chronic pain.

If you are interested in using a topical for your oil needs, make sure that you take some time to read the label. There should be some words like encapsulation, nano-technology, and micellization of the CBD. These will show how the solution is going to carry the CBD through the dermal layers of your skin, providing relief, rather than just having it sit on the skin. This can help you with more issues such as skin or joint concerns.

If you want to use the topical version of the oil, then you just use it the same way that you would use any other skin care product. Test it out on a small area first to see how your skin reacts, and then, if things go well, continue to use it to get the results that you are looking for.

Sprays

Another option that you may want to go with is the sprays. This is not the recommended option to go with because the concentration of the oil is going to be very low. While the other options will be at least 10mg, though they can go higher, the sprays are usually not going to be above 3mg. This makes it hard to get the amount of the oil that you need and can result in you having to take a bunch of it, or not seeing results at all.

But there are a few individuals who decide the spray option is the right one for them. Usually people like these because they can easily carry the spray around with them during the day, and if they just need a low dosage of the product, its quick and easily accessible to use. Remember if you use this option though, it is possible that you will need to use it quite a few times before feeling the effect, and even then the amount may be too low to notice.

Using the spray is pretty easy to work with. To get the full effect, you will just spray one serving of the bottle straight into your mouth and let it sit there for a bit to dissolve. Each spray that you choose to work with is going to have some different rules and servicing sizes. Most will be a serving size of two or three sprays, but always check this before you decide to get started.

Vapes

You can also choose to ingest this oil with the help of vapes. Based on the reviews that some users have left behind for these, they often have fewer effects of the oil when vaping compared to the other options. But then there are also some users who state that they felt better with vaping and they noticed that the side effects were less when they used this method. Honestly, some people have seen a lot of benefits with this method, and others haven't. It is a personal preference if you would like to use this method to help you get the oil.

Edibles

And finally, another option that you may want to choose is edibles. For some people, the taste or the potency or something else of the options that we discussed is not to their liking. For these individuals, edibles could be a nice option. These are baby foods that you can eat that you put the CBD oil inside. You can add CBD to pretty much any snack or meal that you make. Many people like this option because it helps to mask the taste a bit and then you can have a nice snack or meal at the same time. Often the preferred way to do this is to place the oil in a dessert.

While this can be a tastier way to get the oil into your routine, remember that this method is going to take a bit longer to provide you the relief that you want. With other methods, you are absorbing it into the body right away. But with edibles, you have to digest the oil before you get the benefits. This isn't going to be a huge deal, just remember that you are not going to get the benefits as quickly as you will with the other options.

Should I take it with food?

It is usually recommended that you take the oil with some food, or at least not on an empty stomach. If you are using the spray and need to take some while you are on the run in the middle of the day, you will probably be safe since the dosage is so low. But if you are taking a larger dose, or you are taking it right away in the morning, then it may be a good idea to take it, and then eat a good meal afterward.

The reason that this is so important is that the oil can sometimes irritate the stomach if you don't take it with some sort of food. For some people, this is not such a big deal. But for others, it can cause some stomach upsets and can make them feel miserable. To be on the safe side, have some food, or at least a snack when it is time to take the oil.

The best time of day to take?

There really isn't a perfect time of the day to take the CBD oil. Some people like to take it in the morning to alleviate the aches and pains they feel, and others like to wait until the evening so that they can get to sleep at the end of the day. There really isn't a best time of day to take this oil. You can find the time that seems to work the best with the symptoms you are having, and with your own individual schedule.

What dosage should I take

When you are ready to get started with CBD oil, you have to make sure that you take in the right dosage. You want to take enough of the oil to help you see results, but you don't want to take too much either. It can be difficult to know exactly how much you should take since there aren't any official guidelines for this, and most suppliers are going to have their own instructions, which may not be applicable to each person to use it.

Despite the lack of steady guidelines, there are a few things that you can consider when it comes to using

CBD oil for yourself to make sure that you get the right amount. First, there are a few different factors that will come to play when looking at the dosage you should consume. These can include:

1. Your weight
2. The method you use for consuming the oil
3. The strength of the oil
4. The condition you are trying to treat with CBD
5. Your own body chemistry
6. Your age.

The biggest determinant of how much you should take does seem to be based on the condition that you are trying to heal with the oil. There are a few guidelines that you can follow to ensure you get the right dosage of the oil based on whatever condition you are trying to work on:

1. To help fight off any problems with sleeping, you should take between 40 and 160mg a day.

2. To help with epilepsy and other muscle spasm issues, take between 200 and 300 mg a day.
3. To help out with chronic pain, you can take a little bit less, usually between 2 and 20 mg a day.
4. If you have had issues with your appetite after a big illness, one to two mg. a day for a few weeks can help.
5. Some people take the oil to help with schizophrenia. This one is going to have a really big variance and you will have to really experiment with this one to figure out the right dosage. You may need somewhere between 40 and 1280 mg of this each day.
6. To help you deal with some of the mobility issues that come with Huntington's Disease, about 10mg of the oil will help.

There are also some experts that believe you can get the right dosage for this oil based on your weight and the severity of the symptoms that you are dealing with. You can then monitor how that dosage is doing and make any adjustments that you think are needed to keep you healthy. For example, if you weigh 200 pounds and have symptoms that are severe, then you may benefit with taking 30mg of the oil. But for someone who is just 100 pounds with severe issues, they would just take 15 mg. Both would then make adjustments until they find the dosage that works the best for them.

Once you find the dosage of this oil that seems to work the best for you, don't try to increase it. It is tempting to try to increase the amount you take to feel even better, but this doesn't work and for some people, it will actually lessen the effect. This is why it is always best to start with a lower dosage and then work your way up to a higher dosage only if needed.

Things to consider when taking CBD for the first time

For most people, taking CBD oil is a great experience. They start to notice the benefits of the oil almost right away, though the way that you consume it will often determine how long it takes to feel the effects. Even if you aren't taking the oil to help with a particular issue, you will find that this oil can help to give you better sleep at night, helps you to stay focused, and can relieve tension, stress, and muscle aches in no time.

However, it is important to take things slowly when you first get started with this oil. Everyone is going to react differently to this treatment, and sometimes the reactions may not be what you expect. You may feel relaxed enough that it makes driving and basic tasks difficult. You may need to just take things slowly. Some people end up having adverse effects from the oil so it is important to be careful when this happens.

Because it is hard to know how you will react to the oil ahead of time, you may want to consider starting the oil on a few days when you can just be home and relax. Working or driving or doing other strenuous tasks may be difficult when it comes to working with the oil, and until you know how your body is going to behave, it may be best for you to just stay home for the weekend and see how things go. Listen to your body and you will find that you will be able to take the oil without any problems at all.

Chapter 7

THE DIFFERENT STRAINS OF CBD

One thing that many people may not realize about CBD oil is that there are actually many different strains of it. When you begin to do some research about CBD, you will find that you have choices. There isn't just one type that you can pick from; instead, there is a variety and often it will depend on the potency of the mixture. Each strain is going to provide a different kind of relief to the body so you can pick the one that you want to work with based on your symptoms or what you would like it to accomplish. Some of the different strains of CBD oil that you may encounter when you get started includes:

1. Charlotte's Web: If you are looking for a strain of CBD that can help you treat seizures, then Charlotte's web is a great option. It contains only 0.3 percent THC

inside, so the potency that you get will come mainly from the high amount of CBD inside. This strain was actually cultivated to help reduce symptoms in a patient dealing with epilepsy. It was successful and has since grown in popularity because it is a fantastic hemp-based medication, one that can give patients some relief, but still allows you to work, drive, and do other things that are needed in your daily life.

2. Harlequin: Another strain option that you can go with is the Harlequin version. This is going to be an ideal one to go with because of its reliable expression of CBD. It actually comes from a mixture of other strains that are popular, including Colombian Gold, Swiss Landrace, and Thai. Because the ratio is 5:2 between CBD and THC, this is often the strain that is used to treat anxiety and pain. This is also an option to go with if you have trouble consuming the other strains because it offers you a few different

flavorings. For those who are looking for a way to get a break from chronic pain, and a way to relax and effectively deal with anxiety, then this is the best strain to go with.

3. Sour Tsunami: This is a strain that was one of the first to be bred to have a very high amount of CBD chemical in it, rather than having the high THC content. Because it is so high in the CBD chemical, the result is that you get an effective treatment for pain and inflammation, without any bad side effects. In fact, the CBD levels for this strain can be up to 10 percent.

4. Cannatonic: This is a strain that comes to us from Spain. The THC content for this one is going to be below six percent, which is higher than some versions. But what is really impressive is that the CBD content can end up being higher than 17 percent. This is the strain that you will want to use when it is time to relax and mellow out. In addition, it has been used

as a medical treatment for pain, muscle spasms, anxiety, and migraines to name a few.

5. Colombian Gold: This one is actually the basis for a lot of the other strains that we have talked about. It was originally grown in the mountains of Colombia, and the buds are nice and fluffy with a sweet scent that a lot of people tend to enjoy. This strain is one that patients will turn to when they want to reduce their anxiety while also maintaining their productivity all at the same time. It can also relieve pain and muscle tension. It is also the strain that can help the patient feel happier, which makes it a great solution for depression. There is even research that shows how this strain can help patients with ADD and ADHD as well.

6. Sour diesel: This strain is known as one of the more invigorating options out there. It works fast, meaning it won't take a long time before you start to notice the

effects, and it also helps in energizing your brain. If you are dealing with stress, pain, or depression, this can be the strain to help you out. The Sour Diesel strain is also going to last a long time, which makes it the best choice for many medical patients.

7. MK Ultra: This strain is powerful on the brain and can give many patients a hypnotic effect. It is a good medication, especially for patients who find that some of the weaker strains just aren't doing the work. You should be careful because of the strength though and consider just doing it on days when you will have a chance to sit back and relax.

8. Super skunk: This is a strain that will produce a relaxing effect that takes over the body, helping them to calm down and not deal with so much stress or anxiety. The patients who go with this strain find that it is a good one to reduce the levels of stress that they have, and it can help

eliminate aches and pains throughout the body.

9. G13: This is one of those strains that tend to have many urban legends forming around it. Some accounts say that the way this strain was formed was because the CIA and FBI gathered up the very best strains of marijuana in the world and then grew new hybrids out of those. Then a technician took one of the buds from there and released it to others. This particular strain ended up being G13. Of course, it is unlikely that any of these stories are true, but G13 is one of the best strains out there and can help better than medications when it comes to many of the different health conditions you are dealing with.

Each of the strains that we just talked about can be useful when it comes to keeping the body healthy and helping you to get the relief that you need. Choosing the right one will often depend on the type of body ache or other health condition you are trying to work through.

Chapter 8

HEMP OILS

While hempseed oil is seen as a different thing than CBD oil, and true hemp oil is going to be a completely different type of product than the CBD oil that we have talked about, it is important to realize that these two products are often considered to be interchangeable in this industry. In fact, many CBD products are going to be labeled as hemp oils because this allows the suppliers to legally sell them. Hemp oils and hemp seed oils are often seen as legal, while CBD oils are not in most areas. Let's take a look at these hemp oils and how they can be used to help improve your health as well.

Hemp has been cultivated to be used in an industrial setting for many years. In addition to being an oil that can help your body health naturally, it has also been part of the production of paper, rope, cloth, and canvas. These industrial products were, in the past, created with the help of the durable and strong fibers that come with the hemp plant.

However, since hemp is technically from the cannabis plant, this has fueled a lot of confusion and controversy when it comes to products derived from hemp over the years. For some time, the United States made it illegal to even grow hemp, even though it has been used for a very long time just to make common household products. The good news is that the times are changing and hemp is not seen as such a dangerous product any longer.

Today, you will find that there is quite a bit of interest in this hemp oil and how it can work to benefit so many people. While it may be a cool thing to have some of the products made out of hemp, many people don't fully understand how the hemp oil and all of the health benefits that are potentially able to help you out. Let's take a look at some of the things that you should know when it comes to hemp oil and how it compares to CBD oil.

Cannabis use, without having to worry about the high

CBD, or cannabidiol, is actually one of the 113 chemicals that are found in the cannabis plant that are seen as beneficial. While there are some people that might feel a bit uncomfortable when it comes to CBD being a part of the cannabis plant, it should be reassuring that this fact should not cause you any alarm. There are actually two sources for CBD and those include marijuana and hemp.

The CBD that comes from marijuana is going to have a very high level of THC. This level of THC could reach 30 percent or more. Because of this high level of THC, and the fact that this chemical can cause the user to become high, marijuana is now considered a schedule 1 drug in the United States. While the laws that regulate marijuana use are going to be different based on the state you are in, most states are going to consider marijuana as illegal unless you get a prescription for a valid reason from your doctor.

Then it is also possible to extract CBD from hemp. While hemp is part of the cannabis plant, the CBD that is extracted through hemp isn't going to contain the higher levels of THC like what we see with marijuana. There are very clear requirements when it comes to the THC levels the government will accept. To qualify as CBD or hemp oil, the plant needs to have no more than 0.3 percent THC content in it, which is hardly anything.

With a concentration of THC that is that low, it is unlikely that you will ever feel high from taking hemp oil or from taking CBD oil. Even if you take in a huge quantity of either oil. This is great news for many people because it means that the THC won't have a chance to mess or interfere with your motor skills or your cognitive abilities and this means that you can get ahold of hemp oil without having to get permission from a doctor.

CBD oil and Hemp oil are going to be interchangeable.

CBD is known as the abbreviation of cannabidiol, which is one of the biggest and most well-known cannabinoids that are found in the cannabis plant. In addition, when you go online and do a search for hemp sourced CBD product, it is pretty common that you will see hemp oil and CBD oil called the same thing.

Hemp oil is going to contain CBD. It is common that hemp oil and CBD oil are going to be used pretty much as the same thing. Since CBD manufacturers and suppliers are not allowed to include CBD oil on the labels of their products, they are able to choose a label like hemp supplement or hemp oil. Then they will specify the amount of CBD that is in the product to help consumers out. If you are shopping for this product and you see something that goes by hemp oil, take a look to see how much CBD is in it and then determine if it is the option that you are looking for.

CBD doesn't show up in hemp seed oil

While good manufacturers are going to identify their products as hemp oil or CBD oil, it is important to watch out for some of the tricks that shady suppliers may try to use. CBD is going to be a cannabinoid found in the whole plant milled biomass of hemp plants. But when we look at hemp seed oil, this is going to be the oil that is pressed out of the seeds of the plant. What this means is that you are not going to find any CBD inside of hemp seed oil.

When you are taking a look at which products you want to use, you need to really take a look at the ingredients that are found on the label. A good product for CBD is going to specify out the number of milligrams of the CBD which is inside. So, if you are taking a look at a tincture, there may be different potency levels like 250mg or 1000mg in a bottle that is 15 to 30 ml. Capsules are going to be labeled based on the potency of the CBD in each tablet.

If you take a look at the product and notice that the CBD is not specified, then this may mean that the product you are looking at is considered hemp seed oil. The supplier may call it hemp oil or a hemp supplement, but it could easily not have any CBD in it. If there isn't any information on the potency of the product, then it is best to go with something else. Or, if you see a product labeled as hemp seed oil, know that there is absolutely no CBD in it and this isn't the best option if that chemical is what you are looking for.

Methods of getting the CBD out of the hemp

There are several options of extracting the CBD is going to be the same process that is used when you want to create essential oils. There are a few methods that can work, but there are only two that seem to work the best in producing a product that is good for consuming. The two methods below are the best ones to extract CBD out of the hemp plant, and they will ensure that all of the good stuff stays in, while all of the bad stuff stays out.

Looking for products that use one of these two extraction methods is so important to ensure that you get a product that is high quality and will provide you with the results that you want. If another method is used, then this means that contaminants may have gotten into the product, or that something else may be wrong with it.

- ❖ Ethanol extraction: This ethanol is often going to be used as a preservative or an additive to food. The use of this can be a form of chemical extraction. If you use this option with some low temperatures, the ethanol extraction can also help to remove any chlorophyll that is found in the hemp that you wish to remove.

- ❖ CO_2 extraction: This is often seen as the best method to use when extracting CBD oil, and is the one that you should look for in any products you decide to purchase, even though it can cost a bit more. With this method, the supplier will use heavy compression in order to convert the carbon dioxide to a liquid form. This happens with the help of temperature and pressure controlled chambers During this process, the CO_2 is going to dissolve the molecules of the plant, separating all of the other matter of the plant from the oil. The liquid carbon dioxide is then going to convert back to a gaseous state before dispersing and basically cleaning itself up.

CBD and hemp oil are often used interchangeably on the market. And many products that are labeled as hemp oil or hemp supplements go by this name because it makes it easier for the supplier to sell it to their customers. Make sure to check out the amount of CBD that is found in one of these products to ensure that if you choose one, they will provide you with the benefits that you are looking for.

Chapter 9

SIDE EFFECTS

So far in this guidebook, we have talked about some of the great benefits that come with using CBD oil. We looked at the benefits of this kind of medication, the reasons that you should take it, and how it is different compared to marijuana and other cannabis products. With that said, there are times when the oil could cause a few negative reactions or side effects in patients. This is something that is not going to affect every patient, and the majority of the time the oil wont have any side effects at all, which is more than you can say about other medications you may have been prescribed by your doctor in the past.

To get a good idea of how effective CBD oil can be, and to have a full picture of how this substance works, let's take a look at some of the side effects and things that you need to consider before you get started.

Will I experience any side effects?

While there are a lot of great benefits that come with purchasing CBD oil, it is important to realize that some people will experience negative side effects. Often this comes from picking out a supplier who doesn't provide you with the highest quality product, but some people just don't react well to this oil.

The first thing that you need to do is ensure that you do your research and find a reputable seller. This helps you to get a product that is high quality, rather than one that has a lot of other chemicals and additions that may cause you some problems. Always remember that there is no regulation with this oil, so there can be different variations, different names, and more, so you have to always be vigilant to ensure you get the product that you are looking for.

One issue you may encounter with CBD is dry mouth or a sensation of cotton being in the mouth. This may be because the cannabinoid receptors are found in the glands of the mouth, and these ones are going to produce saliva to keep the mouth from getting dry. In some cases, when the oil is introduced, this is going to affect the production of saliva in the mouth, leaving you with a dry feeling there for the first few days. It is not something that is a big danger to your health and usually means that in the beginning, you need to drink a little extra water to counteract the issue.

In some cases, CBD, when taken had higher dosage, is going to result in worsening side effects from the condition that you are trying to treat with the oil. So, those who are using it to deal with muscle tremors may have more issues with their muscles than before, for example. This is why it is important to start out slowly with our consumption of CBD oil and then progress up as needed, and as you can tolerate. Remember that everyone is different. While someone may need a big dosage of the oil, you may be able to get by with just a few drops and see the same results.

In addition, you need to watch the dosage that you are taking because this oil has the ability to stop how a few enzymes in the liver are able to behave. These enzymes are known as the P450 enzymes and they are the ones that will help metabolize the medications that you may already be taking. If you are not careful with the dosage, as we will discuss more in a minute, then this can cause some issues with how effective the medication can be. If you are already on medication before starting this CBD oil, then make sure to discuss the use of it, and how it will affect your current medications, with your doctor right away.

Some of the other side effects that you will need to watch out for include:

- ❖ Lightheadedness: This one ties into the next and often people will feel it because their blood pressure decreases. Try having a cup of tea or some coffee to help get the blood pressure back up, but be careful about the amount that you take each day.
- ❖ Low blood pressure: Taking too much CBD oil for your condition can result in lower blood pressure. This will happen usually right after taking the CBD and you will feel dizzy or lightheaded because of it. This is a

temporary side effect but brings up the point that if you are taking drugs for helping your blood pressure, then you may want to discuss using it, and what dosage is the right one for you, with your doctor before you get started using it.

- ❖ Feeling tired: There are some times when this treatment can cause drowsiness, but again, this usually happens when the dosage of CBD is high. If you do happen to feel drowsy when taking it, you need to be careful when driving or using machinery and may need to consider reducing your dosage. In most cases, as long as the dosage is appropriate for the person, it will actually work to help you feel full of energy and more awake, rather than inducing sleep.

How will I know I am having a negative reaction?

It is important to listen to your body when you are ready to start out with this kind of oil. It is generally thought to be safe for most individuals to use, but in some instances, it could end up causing serious health issues, especially for those who are on medications. This is why it is important to take things slow and start with a lower dosage. This allows you a chance to see how your body will react so you can make adjustments, without causing harm to your body.

If you are on medication and notice that there is an increase in the symptoms that you have for your medical condition, then it is time to stop taking the oil. CBD can sometimes make the matter worse because it will change up the way your body takes in the medication. If your body eats up the medication and then disperses it into the body at a different rate than usual, it is possible that your symptoms will get worse, and this means it is time to stop.

If you notice that you feel more side effects from the medication you take when you also take CBD oil, then it is time to stop taking the oil. Sometimes the side effects that come with CBD are going to be similar to what you get from the medications you are on. If these side effects all occur at the same time, things are going to get. If this happens, you should stop taking the CBD oil and talk to your doctor about this issue.

Of course, there are times when you may take the oil on its own without any other medications. If you are doing this and notice that your dry mouth is becoming excessive, then it is time to stop. This can definitely be a problem if you decided to try the oil in order to increase your appetite to help gain weight. Having a mouth that is really dry all the time can make eating even more difficult, which is not only uncomfortable but makes the work of the oil pretty ineffective to start with.

Be careful about your blood pressure going down too much as well. This can result in issues like dizziness, lightheadedness, and even fainting in some extreme cases. This can sometimes happen when you get up too fast from either sitting or laying down, though some people claim it can happen even when they stay still. If this is something that happens to you while taking the CBD oil, then it is time to stop taking it.

And finally, if you are taking the oil and find that you are feeling really drowsy, enough that you doze off frequently and you often feel confused, then it is time to stop this medication and consult your doctor on what you should do next. If you feel this way, don't drive, cook, or take care of children because your state of awareness is not fully there. Usually, the oil is going to make you more attentive and alert so feeling incredibly drowsy is not a good sign at all.

Should I see a doctor before starting?

For most patients, it is perfectly safe to get started on CBD oil. You will notice a dramatic change in your symptoms and you will start to feel better than ever before. You can safely experiment a bit with your CBD oil consumption and not have to worry about getting sick or running into any of the negative side effects that we have been talking about.

But for some individuals, it may be better to discuss the use of these oils with your doctor before you get started. Individuals who are on blood thinners, have seizures, or are on other medications may need to talk to their doctor beforehand. This ensures that they understand how the oil will affect them while they are on their other medications, and can allow you some time to discuss any questions or concerns before you get started. If there is a serious reason why you shouldn't take CBD oil, your doctor will be able to discuss this with you as well.

Do medications and CBD oils mix?

If you are already taking some medications for a variety of health conditions, it is important to consider whether starting CBD oil is the best choice for you. Often we don't want to go completely off our current medications because we aren't sure how we will react with them, and we may not be sure about how we will react to the CBD oil. But, is it really safe to mix our current medications with the CBD oil that we want to try out?

One of the biggest downfalls of working with CBD is that there hasn't been as much research done on it as there should be. This is especially true when it comes to how this oil is going to potentially interact with other drugs. CBD, even though safe and effective, is a chemical compound that is going to have a specific effect on the different pathways in the body. This is why it is so important to know whether these effects are going to be counterproductive or even dangerous when you take them along with some other substances.

The good news is that the research that is out there, along with testimonials from other, have found that it is now widely accepted that this oil is going to be safe to use in most cases, even when you take it with other medications. In one study that was published in 2017, it was confirmed that it is safe to take CBD with other medications and even proved that doing this had a better side effect profile when it was compared to medications that were supposed to act in a similar manner.

In addition, the U.S. Department of Health also issued a statement in the past few years that claimed that "series adverse effects are rare with cannabis or its constituents."

With that being said, there have been several smaller studies that show that if you take larger doses of CBD, the oil has the ability to inhibit and even deactivate one of the enzymes in the liver, the one that is important for efficiently breaking down prescription medications that the individual needs to take. If these medications are not broken down in a timely manner, the accumulation of them can be dangerous and that is going to allow for a stagnant buildup of compounds in the liver, and an intense effect of the drug on the person.

While there needs to be more research done on how well CBD oil can interact with some of the other medications that you may consider taking, some of the most common medications that have been studied so far include:

1. Blood thinners: Heparin and Warfarin are subject to a longer activity, and even an increased effect when they are taken at the same time as the oil. This means that if you are taking a blood thinner at the time, you need to be extra careful about the frequency and the dosage of the oil. You may want to discuss the use of this with your doctor beforehand.

2. Medications to help with peptic ulcers and reflux: Omeprazole, which can include some other drugs like Losec and Prilosec, can also be affected if you use CBD on a regular basis. In fact, the effect of these medications can be blocked if a significant dose of the oil is taken before you take the other medications.
3. Medications that help with autism, bipolar, and schizophrenia: Medications like Risperidone are often going to be blocked and ineffective when they are used along with the CBD oil.
4. Cholesterol medications: If you take in frequent amounts of the CBD, it could help increase the serum concentration of many cholesterol-lowering drugs.
5. Medications for blood pressure: While CBD may not be known to increase the levels of your blood pressure, the combination of CBD and THC together has sometimes initiated cardiac stress responses and can reduce the arterial blood flow. If you are taking any

medication to help with blood pressure, you must be aware that taking this kind of oil could enhance the effects of your medication. Depending on the results, this could cause some serious complications.

6. Epilepsy and seizure medications: It is believed that CBD oil can help lessen the effects of epilepsy and seizures in many patients. But for those who are already on medication for those conditions, it is important to be careful.

While there are a ton of great benefits that come with using CBD oil on a daily basis, it is important to realize that there are also some side effects that can't be ignored either. Understanding the side effects, and when to get off the oil can be key to keeping your health in the best shape.

Chapter 10

Myths and Mistakes

As we know, there is a lot of information out there that talks about CBD oil. Some of the information is going to help you learn more about the product, how to use it, and all of the great benefits that come with this product and how it can improve your life. But as the popularity of this product grows, there are also a lot of sites that will spread misinformation and myths about the product as well.

Before you decide to get started with the CBD oil, it is important to dispel these myths so that you are on the right page when you try to get your results. This chapter is going to dispel some of the common myths that are out there about CBD oil, while also discussing some of the biggest mistakes beginners make when they start that you should avoid, so you can get the most out of your experience with CBD oil.

Common myths about CBD oil

While CBD has been around for a number of years, there are still a lot of myths and common misconceptions out there about this product. Many people in the Western world know very little about cannabis, and thanks to the DEA, many of us only know about marijuana and that it is considered illegal. But CBD is different. It can provide us with so many great health benefits that can improve all aspects of our lives. To help you make a decision on whether CBD oil is the right choice for you or not, let's look at some common myths about this product and why they just aren't true.

The oil isn't safe for children

There are some parents who are naturally hesitant to let their children take this oil. Because there is a widespread misunderstanding of CBD oil and how it is different from cannabis. These parents worry that giving this oil to their child will result in them getting high and having other serious side effects. But true CBD oil comes from the hemp plant. It may be a type of cannabis plant, but what many people don't realize is the THC which causes the usual negative side effects of taking cannabis, is less than 0.3 percent. CBD is non-psychoactive and in fact, could negate some of the psychoactive effects of THC, making it perfectly safe for children.

All products with CBD in them are the same

Because there are no regulations on this industry, all CBD products are not going to be the same. Each supplier can choose to create and sell the products in a different manner, which is why the consumer needs to pay attention and do their research before they decide to make a purchase. Just like many other products you may want to purchase on the market, some of these are going to be higher quality compared to others.

The quality of these products is often going to depend on where the supplier got the CBD from. There are many origins for this chemical, but the highest quality ones usually come from Europe or the United States. Purchasing a product that comes from one of these two areas can really help you to get one of the best products out there.

You may find as you do your research that figuring out which businesses are legitimate can be hard as well. There are no regulations so you have to know what you are looking for, even as a beginner. This is why it is a great idea to check out whether the company uses third-party lab testing. This allows you to see that a testing agency, one that isn't associated with the business, has checked out the product and verifies it is of good quality and will work. The fact that a company has spent extra money for this testing, and published the results, is a good sign that they want to provide you with a good product.

CBD is considered a sedative

While it is true that certain dosages of CBD can help you get a better nights' sleep because it helps get rid of some of the anxiety and pain that keeps you up at night, this chemical is not a sedative by itself. And since CBD can help to dampen some of the THC sedation, it actually works in the opposite way, providing you more energy to say awake and have energy.

Many of those who decide to go on CBD find that they actually feel more alert when they take this oil, and they also find it even truer when especially taking large doses of the oil. For others, the larger doses can calm them down a bit, especially if they are already dealing with anxiety, and this helps them to sleep better than before. Either way, CBD is going to provide you with a way to sleep better, but this is because it relaxes the body and can get rid of a lot of pain that you may feel, rather than causing you to go into sedation.

You have to take a large amount of CBD to get results

As more and more people start to learn about CBD, there are going to be more suppliers who enter the market and provide products infused with CBD. They may even provide more methods to receive the chemical besides the ones we talked about before. The biggest problem that can come with these products is that since there are no regulations on them, they will contain a varying amount of CBD. Some can contain just a few milligrams a serving, and others will have hundreds of milligrams in each serving.

Depending on the dosage that is right for you, and the condition you are trying to fix, the large milligram amounts in a serving will be too much to provide you with any benefits. When the individual takes these larger amounts and then doesn't see any benefits (which will often happen when they take too much), they will usually assume that the CBD is ineffective and that it does not work for them.

Everyone is different and there may be some people who do need to take a larger dose of the oil to see results. But then there are some who could get away with a much lower dose and still see results. If you start out with 500 mg a day, it is hard to tell if you are getting enough or too little of the product, because the results will be the same. Most people don't need a large amount of this chemical to feel better, so starting out small and building up is the best way to get to the right dosage and to get the benefits promised.

Hemp CBD oil and hemp seed oil are the same

This is a sneaky little trick that some suppliers like to use to sell a product to unsuspecting customers who haven't done their research. Hemp seed oil does not have any CBD in it at all. It may have some valuable nutrients depending on how the supplier processes it, but you won't get the same benefits as you will from CBD oil. Always be sure to be to look for hemp CBD oil and not just hemp oil when looking to buy this product, so you can gain the benefits we have talked about previously, and not waste money.

If you see a supplier offering hemp seed oil, stay away from these altogether. Sometimes they will be priced lower, but some unscrupulous suppliers tend to decide to sell it at the same or even a higher price than regular hemp CBD oils. You won't be able to get the same results if you pick these though because they are definitely not the same thing, regardless of what the supplier is telling you.

There isn't any evidence that CBD provides all these good benefits

As you have read in this guidebook, there are a ton of benefits that you can get when you decide to add CBD into your life. And there are studies to help back it up. While the studies are still pretty new, there are just so many benefits that come with this chemical that it is hard to have time to conduct that much research so far. This doesn't mean there isn't any research to look into the effects.

In fact, there is a ton of research out there. For almost every ailment that CBD oil is claimed to help with, there are at least one or two studies done, even though some of them are short term studies. As more people start to use this oil for their health, and the use takes place over a longer term, more studies will come out to prove these great benefits.

Mistakes you should avoid when taking this oil?

As someone who is new to the world of CBD oil, it is common to have a lot of questions and concerns that you want to deal with right from the beginning. No one wants to spend time working with these products and then finding out that they have made mistakes or they are using the product in the wrong manner. Some of the most common mistakes that you should avoid when it comes to taking CBD oil include the following:

Assuming that this oil will get you high

As we have discussed in this guidebook, CBD oil is never going to get you high. THC is the main active component of cannabis and marijuana that will get you the effect of being high. While there is a tiny bit of THC in the CBD oil, the amounts that are allowed in these products is so low, that you could drink the oil all day long and never feel high.

The whole point of taking these products is to help improve various other aspects of your health. Many people have fallen in love with the CBD oil because it has helped to improve their health and their lives so much, all without the feelings of being high and the negative side effects that come from that.

Setting up unrealistic expectations

There are so many things that this CBD oil can help you with. Such things like helping to protect your heart, having the potential to prevent and fight cancer, lowering blood pressure, helping with acne, treating symptoms of depression and anxiety, and even reduce inflammation. The list of benefits that come with CBD oil seems to be endless, and so many people are just jumping on and giving it a try.

While CBD oil can be efficient at helping out with a ton of different conditions, it is important to remember that your expectations about this oil must be realistic. While there may be some relief from the symptoms you are dealing with, it isn't going to happen overnight. You may need to experiment with the dosage for some time, and try out a few different times of day to consume the oil. You may find that it takes a few weeks to even see some noticeable results.

In addition, there are some people who will go on this oil with the assumption that after a few weeks, they will be able to reduce their medications and still feel good. This is possible for some conditions and for some people, but it doesn't always happen. Expecting this from the beginning, without a good idea of how the body will react to the oil at all, can set you up for disappointment.

Instead of feeling this way, it is much better to just make the goal of feeling better when you take the oil.

If you start out with this and aim towards finding a dosage that can give you your health back, even a little, then you are going to be more impressed with the results.

Choosing affordability over quality

This is really one place where you shouldn't go for the cheapest option on the market. Sure, everyone wants to save money wherever possible, but the cheapest CBD oils on the market are going to contain a lot of extra additives that could cause harm, may have a higher level of THC than recommended, could be heavily diluted, or may have some other problems with them.

When it comes to using CBD oil, it is best to find quality instead of affordability. Otherwise, your only risking potential issues with a product that doesn't work because it doesn't actually contain the chemicals that you are looking for, or at least doesn't contain them in the concentrations that you believe. When you are searching for a good CBD product to go with, make sure that you look for quality and then find a good deal from there.

Not taking things slowly

While CBD and hemp oils are seen as relatively safe, each person is going to react to it differently. Even if you start out with a lower dosage of the product, it is important that for at least the first few days, you take things slowly and see how they go. Sometimes you will feel tired and drowsy, may have an upset stomach or other problems that can make you uncomfortable. Taking the oil on a day when you can just be at home and relax a bit, at least the first few times that you take it, can be key to getting yourself used to it.

Using the wrong method

There are a variety of different methods that you can use, but not all of them will be as effective as others. You need to pick out the method that makes the most sense for you, the one that helps you to get the oil in the most effective way possible, and one that works for the condition that you want to heal. Most people find that working with sublingual options is the most effective, but if you can't stand the flavor or can't make that option work, you then need to choose from some of the other options to get the results.

Not researching the supplier you use

Always take the time to do some research on the supplier that you wish to use. There are a lot of suppliers out there, and many of them are going to provide you with a product that is high quality and will give you the benefits that you are looking for. But because of the profitability of these products and this industry, there are also going to be some companies and suppliers who will sell a substandard or bad product, and you will be the one paying the price in the end.

Some suppliers know how to work around the wording of their products in order to make them look good and to convince you to purchase them. Always take a look at the THC content in each product, determine the CBD concentration in the products, and look out if a product states that it is hemp seed oil. Look at the reviews of the seller and check how other customers have faired with using this company. Also look to see where the product offered by the supplier has been tested by a third party lab.

Not experimenting to find the right dosage

When you first get ahold of the CBD oil, you are probably excited to get started. You have heard a lot of good things about this oil and you are excited to see how the benefits can affect you. You want to jump right into using the product without having to worry about slowly testing the waters and finding your perfect dosage. Maybe you already know someone else who has taken this oil in the past, or who currently is, and you think that you should just take the same amount that they do.

But no matter what, it is important to experiment and try to find the right dosage for you. Each person is going to be different and the way that a friend reacted to the treatment may be different compared to the way that you respond to it. Taking too much of the oil can have the same effect as taking too little of it, and if you start out with a high amount, it is hard to tell if you have had too much, or if the treatment isn't effective for you.

A much better option to go with is starting out with the minimum recommended amount based on the condition that you are trying to deal with. If you find that amount is not right, then you slowly add in more to your routine. Once you start to feel an alleviation to the symptoms you were suffering from, this is a good place to stop. If you keep going, you may find that the symptoms come back because your dosage is too high. Go back down to the amount that made you feel good, and stick with that.

Experimenting with your dosage can be so important to ensure that you are going to see the best results. It helps you to learn how your body reacts to the oil and can help you to make the adjustments that are right for you. Each person is going to be different. Some people can take smaller dosages of the oil compared to others, and that is fine. But finding your perfect amount is critical to seeing the success that you want.

Chapter 11

Legality of CBD Oil

Knowing now the full effects and benefits of CBD oil, you may also be wondering if it is legal to sell, produce, buy, or possess the oil at all. This chapter is going to take a look at some of the legal aspects of CBD oil you may be concerned about before you decide to get started with it.

Are CBD and hemp oils legal?

The first thing to explore here is whether or not CBD oil or hemp oils are actually legal. While there are a ton of great health benefits that come from CBD oil, and we already spent some time talking about them in this guidebook, there are still many questions from current and potential users about whether it is actually legal to use these oils for that purpose.

The issue here is that CBD kind of falls into a grey area of the law. While this oil is not technically the same as marijuana because it doesn't contain the THC, it does come from the same part of the cannabis plant. And this is where the issue is going to occur.

In both the United States and the United Kingdom, as well as with a lot of other western countries, there isn't going to be any differences between the parts of the cannabis plant. They see the plant as a whole and they have made it illegal to possess and use that plant in any form. All of the products that come off that plant and any of the ways that you would use them are technically going to be seen as illegal.

So this brings up the question of if you sell or purchase the CBD oil, are you doing something that is illegal and will you get in trouble for doing either of these things, despite all of the good benefits?

For years, the reason that CBD oil was a thriving business that did well was that there was a bit of ambiguity that showed up in the Federal Controlled Substances Act and the way it decided to define marijuana. In the past, there wasn't any inclusion of the mature stalks of the plant. These mature stalks are the part that will make up hemp. Therefore, hemp is technically not illegal because the part of the plant that was used to create it isn't covered under the legal definition of marijuana.

To take this further, the CBD oil, at least the part that is non-psychoactive, is made with the use of hemp rather than using the rest of the plant. Since the parts that were used to make hemp were legal, many manufacturers were able to use this as a way to legally produce CBD oil without an issue, even in areas where marijuana was illegal.

This issue also grew more in 2014 with the Farm Bill. This was the Bill that allowed for some manufacturers to cultivate hemp, as long as they were able to keep the THC levels lower than 0.3 percent. Since this is the level of most of the CBD oils that you will find (and some even lower), it made it easier for manufacturers and even suppliers of this chemical to sell their products and still remain legal in their operations.

However, things are not always as simple as they seem. Even though both of these bills seem to point to the fact that CBD oil should be legal, this is still considered a bit of a grey area in many cases. Since marijuana is considered a controlled substance and is found to not be legal in most states in the country, it is important to be careful. There are some loopholes that come with it, but technically, since all the parts of the cannabis plant are illegal, technically the CBD oil, no matter what kind, would be considered illegal as well.

Because of the confusion that comes between the legal definition of marijuana and some of the other bills that have been passed since that time, the Drug Enforcement Administration decided in 2016 to address this issue. This was meant to help avoid any technicalities that may show up and would let people know whether they were on the right side of the law with the products or not. The DEA basically released regulations that made it impossible for manufacturers of CBD oil to work around the new definition of marijuana with the introduction of the Controlled Substance Act.

With these new rules in place, there is now a code number in place for Controlled Substances that is set aside to provide information on extracts of marijuana. The point of doing this code number is to extend out the classification of marijuana to extracts that have one or more cannabinoids from any plant of the genus Cannabis. If you remember from before, or from other research, since CBD is considered a cannabinoid and hemp comes from the genus Cannabis, this means that most products that have CBD in them, whether they are sold online or in a store, are going to fit under this new regulation.

But the DEA decided to take this a little bit further. Instead of just writing out the new code about CBD oil, they also confirmed that "For practical purposes, all extracts that contain CBD oil will also contain just small amounts of other cannabinoids. However, if it were possible to produce from the cannabis plant an extract that contained only CBD, such an abstract would now fall within the new drug code 7350."

This is meant to make sure that there are no loopholes to the system and that everyone is on the same page when it comes to whether CBD and hemp oil are seen as something legal in the country or not. The reason that the DEA went to such efforts for this new rule is to ensure that the United States was able to comply with the UN Convention on Narcotic Drugs. It was also a way to make sure that the various suppliers weren't going to be able to dance around the various loopholes that had been used in the previous bills.

So, what is this going to mean for the suppliers as well as the sellers of various CBD products, whether they are doing it online or they are doing it in states that don't have the most progressive laws on cannabis? While there is a lot of legal and flowery words that show up around the definition, the DEA is telling everyone that CBD oil and other similar products are now illegal when you look under the Controlled Substances Act. Even though it is made and used differently, and it doesn't have the same chemicals inside of it, CBD oil is going to be treated the same way as other cannabinoids are. This is something that law enforcement recognized before, but now it can be enforced on sellers when they are caught thanks to the DEA.

Of course, this doesn't mean that all hope is lost. There are a lot of sellers out there who can still grow and sell these kinds of products, despite the fact that the DEA is hardening up their laws concerning this product. Most of the sellers are going to be in areas, such as Colorado, where cannabis is considered legal. This allows them to do the work in a completely legal way.

However, if you don't live in one of those areas, you need to be especially careful if you decide to go with one of these products. Even if you order the product from Colorado, or some other state when they open up and legalize marijuana and cannabis. If you live in another state like Nebraska, then you can still get into trouble if someone catches you with the substance.

This doesn't mean that the laws are stuck that way and won't ever be able to change. There has already been a big movement to legalize marijuana and the other parts of the cannabis plant, and much of this is due to the fact that many people are starting to see some of the benefits that come with this chemical. As more and more people learn about CBD and the other non-toxic and helpful chemicals that come from this plant, it is more likely that these laws can be changed.

Still, you must realize what the laws are when it comes to these products, and there could be some issues when you decide to purchase these products. Be aware of the issues if you live in a state where cannabis, in all of its forms, is still considered illegal. But if you live in a state, or even a country, where cannabis is not illegal, and you get the product from a seller who is from an area where it is legal, then you will be good to go.

Can I fail a drug test taking CBD oil?

Let's say that you have been taking CBD oil for a little bit of time. You grew some of your own or got it from someone who produced it in a state where it is legal. But you may live in an area where this oil is not considered legal at all. While CBD oil is considered non-toxic, it still falls on the wrong side of the law, and it is natural to be worried about who could find out that you are using this option for your health.

The answer to this is going to depend on your suppliers. A pure form of CBD oil is going to be so low in THC, that the numbers would never show up on a urine drug test. This means if your supplier did a good job, you can use the CBD oil and no one would be able to find it on a drug test.

However, if your supplier was not careful with how well they removed the THC, or you pick out one of the CBD oil strains that have higher levels of THC, then this is going to show up in the drug test that you do. It all depends on the strain that you use, how much THC is found in that strain, and how careful your supplier was to start with.

The safest bet, even if you trust your supplier and you went with a strain that had a lower THC content in it, is to try to avoid taking the product for at least a few days before a known drug test. This will ensure that the THC has time to pass through the body before you have to take the test so that nothing shows up when you take it.

Is it legal to grow and make your own CBD oil?

In the United States, it is still largely illegal to grow hemp to make CBD oil. However, there have been a few states recently that have tried to change this up a bit, and this has allowed more sellers and manufacturers to provide this valuable product to their consumers. North Dakota, California, Vermont, and Colorado have all passed laws that enable hemp licensure, which can allow certain companies or individuals to start producing their own help and creating the CBD oil that so many people want. If you live in one of the other states in the country though, it is still considered illegal to grow and make hemp, which in turn makes it illegal to make your own CBD oil.

There are a number of other western countries who have legal hemp growing in them. Some of these include:

- ❖ New Zealand and Australia: These allow for some research crops.

- ❖ Canada: In 1994, Canada started to license some research crops to see how it would go. Then by 1997, many acres of the plant where done. Canada now provides licenses for commercial agriculture of the product.
- ❖ Most of Europe: Hemp growing is legal in most of Europe including countries such as Denmark, Finland, France, Germany, Great Britain, Hungary, Poland, Switzerland and the Netherlands.

Is it legal to sell?

This is going to depend on where you live. In certain countries, and even in certain states in the United States, you are allowed to legally grow and sell marijuana. If you reside in one of these states, then you can go ahead and sell your own CBD oil all that you want. Some people in these areas choose to just make enough so they can use it for personal use to help treat the symptoms that they have, whilst others choose to make a lot more to sell at a profit.

Even when it comes to living in a state where cannabis is legal, you have to be careful. The laws are often changing and with federal pressure running high, it is possible that the laws could change quickly, and the legality of your actions could be called into question. At this current time though, you should be pretty safe to continue on with this process, just make sure that you are always staying up to date on your local news to see if any changes occur.

Another thing to consider is who you sell the products to. It is perfectly legal if you sell some of the product to someone who is in the same state as you. But if you try to send the product out of state, there can sometimes be issues with the legality of it. Many sellers have sent out products to different parts of the country, including to states where cannabis is not legal. But you have to be aware that this could run you into some legal trouble as well.

If you live in a state or a country were cannabis is considered illegal, then it is definitely not legal for you to sell. If you have a small crop to help you get the CBD oil to treat your own conditions, then this may be something you can get away with. If you are uncertain, consider getting a doctor's note for this treatment. But once you start trying to sell the product in these areas, you are going to run into the wrong side of the law.

The legal aspects that come with CBD oil can be kind of murky. The DEA has changed up some of the rules, which has made it harder for some suppliers to provide the product to their customers. But then there are many states that have now legalized cannabis in all of its forms, which has helped to open this up a bit more again. Figuring out what the law says about each of these can be a hard thing to work with.

Conclusion

Thanks for making it through to the end of CBD and Hemp Oil, let's hope it was informative and able to provide you with all of the tools you need to achieve your goals whatever they may be.

The next step is to start looking for your supply of CBD oil so you can start seeing the benefits that you want. This guide not only spent some time discussing the great benefits that you can get when working with the CBD oil, but we also spent time looking at the different ways that you can take the oil, where to find a good supplier, the different dosages that are recommended, and so much more. Keep this guide with you to ensure you get the best results with your CBD consumption possible!

Finally, if you found this book useful in anyway, a review is always appreciated!

Description

Have you ever been curious about CBD oil? Have you heard a lot of talk about this oil, talk that sounds like it could be the answer to your health issues, and you want to learn more? CBD oil is taking the world by storm, providing relief from many serious health conditions, without causing all of the negative side effects that we are used to seeing in the traditional medications we get to deal with these conditions. This guidebook will take some time to look more in-depth at CBD oil and discuss everything you need to know to get started.

This guidebook is going to cover all of the aspects that you need to know about CBD oil including:

- ❖ What is CBD oil and Hemp oil and how are they different and the same
- ❖ How CBD oil is able to help you alleviate your aches and pains.
- ❖ Using these oils to help fight off depression and anxiety.
- ❖ Other health benefits of these oils.

- ❖ Some of the essentials that you need to know when you purchase these oils.
- ❖ The different methods of consuming these oils and how to get to get the dosage right.
- ❖ Some of the different strains of CBD that you can find and choose from.
- ❖ Hemp oils and how they are different than CBD oil.
- ❖ The side effects that you should watch for when taking these oils.
- ❖ Common mistakes and myths that come with CBD consumption
- ❖ Understanding the legality of using CBD oil for your health.

The world of medicine is changing, and relying on expensive and harmful medications is a thing of the past. When you are ready to learn more about CBD oil and all that it has to offer for your health, make sure that you check out this guidebook to help you get started.